This Book is the Property of

_____

The Intermittent Fasting Diet Food Diary
The Ultimate Diet Log
Jean LeGrand

Copyright © 2014 FastForward Publishing All rights reserved. Permission to reproduce or transmit in any form or by any means, electronic or mechanical, including photocopying and recording, or by any information storage or retrieval system, must be obtained in writing from FastForward Publishing.

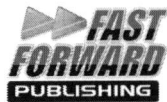

FastForwardPublishing.com

ISBN-13: 978-1505785210
ISBN-10: 1505785219

Table of Contents

Introduction	3
Why Keep a Food Log?	4
How to Use This Food Log	5
A Word about Intermittent Fasting	8
Final Thoughts	9
Your Food Log	10
Bonus	138
FastForward Journals	139
About The Author	140

Before starting any new diet, it is recommended that you discuss the diet and your approach to it with your primary care doctor.

Introduction

Most of us are unaware of our eating habits, and it's that lack of top-of-mind awareness that contributes to our inability to lose weight or to make dietary adjustments to improve our health like reducing our vulnerability to illnesses like heart disease and diabetes.

Do you know how many sodas you drink in a month? On average, how many daily servings of green, leafy vegetables do you typically eat in a week? I could go on, but the point is: If you don't know what your habits are, how are you going to change them?

Why Keep a Food Log?

Keeping a food log has been proven to one of the most effective tools for people to make lifestyle choices in regard to healthy consumption of food.

One reason for this is people typically do not really know much about their food consumption; research has established that there's a huge discrepancy between what we eat and what we think we eat. According to a Cornell University study, 5 minutes after eating a meal at an Italian restaurant, the diners thought they ate 30% less bread than what the hidden cameras showed them actually eating.

The majority of people firmly believe that they eat far more nutritiously than they actually do. A food log shows the difference between what we think we eat and what we actually eat, setting the stage for us to change our habits for the better.

There are many studies that have shown that people who keep food journals are more likely to be successful in losing weight and keeping it off. In a six month study published in the *American Journal of Preventive Medicine,* people keeping a food diary six days a week lost about twice as much weight as those who kept food records one day a week or less.

How to Use This Food Log

This food log has been designed for flexibility; you don't have to fill out every single area marked if you don't want to. That being said, try to be consistent so when you review your entries over a week or month or longer, you have information that can help you understand how you eat and how you are (or should be) changing your relationship with food.

Step 1: Determine Your Reasons

If you are going to commit to this process, be clear on your intent, so you will collect meaningful information to address your specific concern. Here are some typical reasons that people choose to keep a food log followed by what information they should be recording in the log:

Nutrition: along with recording the food and beverage consumed, enter in the nutritional components (fat, sugar, salt, etc.).

Portions: along with recording the food and beverage consumed, focus on recording the weight and measurement of those things you eat.

Emotional Eating: along with entering the food and beverage consumed, record your moods and note possible connections to eating patterns.

Health: track those aspects of diet that impact your particular concern. Keeping track of carbs, fat, and fiber grams will be helpful for people with diabetes and other medical conditions. For example, if you have type 2 diabetes, you might discover that your blood sugar levels improve when your meal or snack contains a certain amount of fiber.

Habitual Eating Patterns: along with entering the food and beverage consumed, focus on recording the time of day, the location, people with whom you ate, and any activity that was taking place while you ate.

Step 2: Commit to a Level of Detail

Maybe you're not ready (or the type of person) to fill out a detailed food log form each day. No problem; even the process of just jotting down a minimum amount of information in your food diary will help you self-monitor.

Don't worry about perfection. You haven't failed because you miss a detail or two. Remember that every attempt you make at recording gets you a step closer realizing the benefits of paying attention to food choices and habits.

> NOTE: Experts say it's important to record everything – even if it makes you uncomfortable. Although it is tempting to skip recording that unplanned dessert, it is important that you write it down and review it as part of your understanding of how to improve your relationship with food.

Step 3: Decide How Often to Update

For the best results, you should write in your food log every day. At a minimum you should write in it at 5 days a week.

The experts say your record (and, thus your results) will be more accurate if you write in your food log immediately after eating.

We've made this food log a small enough size (6" x 9") that you should be able to easily carry it with you and fill it out as you go throughout the day. If that's not feasible for you, set some time aside at the end of the day to update it.

> NOTE: As time goes on, people typically tend to become more complacent and lax about how often they update their food logs and wait a longer period of time after

eating or drinking before logging the information. Try to avoid this trap.

Step 4: Beware of Success Inhibitors

Research shows us that the 5 most common obstacles to keeping a food log are:

> A person is embarrassed or ashamed about their eating
>
> A person has a sense of hopelessness, feeling that it won't help to fill out a food log
>
> A person feels that weight loss is impossible for them
>
> It seems daunting and inconvenient to a person to write down what they eat/drink
>
> A person feels bad when they "slip up"

How do you deal with these obstacles? Sherrie Delinsky, PhD, a staff psychologist at Massachusetts General Hospital, suggests: *"All of these obstacles can be overcome by remembering the usefulness of the diaries, not trying to be perfect, acknowledging that slips will happen, and staying motivated to use tools that promote health and well-being."*

A Word About Intermittent Fasting

According to *U.S. News & World Report,* the theory behind it is that our bodies were programmed for periods of feast and famine. As such, we should recreate these feast and famine days in order to lose weight and live a longer life.

On this plan (also called The Fast Diet), dieters select two non-consecutive days each week to eat 500 or 600 calories, depending if they're a man or woman. On fasting days, low-glycemic-index and low-glycemic-load foods are recommended since they take longer to digest, which in turn makes you feel more satisfied. Recommended foods include vegetables, nuts, seeds, legumes (including beans and lentils), and some fruit. Dieters are recommended to follow their regular exercise regimen during fasting days. During the remaining five non-fasting days, you can eat whatever you wish.

Final Thoughts

You are taking an important step in a journey that will shed light on the way you approach food. You are going to gather information that will help you become healthier as you develop good nutritional habits.

This is not the toughest task you've ever set for yourself, but it will have its challenging moments. Just remember to stick with it even when you are not totally motivated. And if you miss a day or two, don't give up, remember those things inspired you to start in the first place and get re-started without "beating yourself up".

Also, be honest. It's a journal, not a newsletter. No one has to see it but you; and the more honest you are, the bigger the positive impact on your life.

You're taking action. Good for you. Celebrate the little victories along with the big ones. Feel good about completing a day. Get pumped about completing a week. Be proud of getting back to the log after missing a day or two.

And most of all, embrace the idea you are doing something good for yourself, and that you deserve it.

"Developing a diet that is healthful, balanced, and
appropriate for your particular caloric needs
is easy enough and is absolutely critical
to establishing a healthful lifestyle
that incorporates proper nutrition,
adequate fitness, and
mental resilience."

Daphne Oz

Daily Food Log   Day:_____   Date:_____

Hours of Sleep Last Night: ☐ 0-2   ☐ 2-4   ☐ 4-6   ☐ 6-8   ☐ 8-10   ☐ 10+

# of 8 oz. glasses of water consumed: ☐ ☐ ☐ ☐ ☐ ☐ ☐ ☐ ☐ ☐

Vitamins, Supplements, Medications:

Breakfast	Calories	Protein	Carbs	Fiber	Fat	Added Sugar
Time: Totals:						

Mid-Morning Snack	Calories	Protein	Carbs	Fiber	Fat	Added Sugar
Time: Totals:						

Lunch	Calories	Protein	Carbs	Fiber	Fat	Added Sugar
Time: Totals:						

Mid-Afternoon Snack	Calories	Protein	Carbs	Fiber	Fat	Added Sugar
Time: Totals:						

Dinner	Calories	Protein	Carbs	Fiber	Fat	Added Sugar
Time: Totals:						

Evening Snack	Calories	Protein	Carbs	Fiber	Fat	Added Sugar
Time: Totals:						

Daily Totals	Calories	Protein	Carbs	Fiber	Fat	Added Sugar
Totals for all Meals and Snacks:						

Fitness Activity   Time   Duration

_____

_____

Daily Food Log   Day:_____   Date:_____

Hours of Sleep Last Night: ☐ 0-2   ☐ 2-4   ☐ 4-6   ☐ 6-8   ☐ 8-10   ☐ 10+

# of 8 oz. glasses of water consumed: ☐ ☐ ☐ ☐ ☐ ☐ ☐ ☐ ☐ ☐

Vitamins, Supplements, Medications:

Breakfast	Calories	Protein	Carbs	Fiber	Fat	Added Sugar
Time: Totals:						

Mid-Morning Snack	Calories	Protein	Carbs	Fiber	Fat	Added Sugar
Time: Totals:						

Lunch	Calories	Protein	Carbs	Fiber	Fat	Added Sugar
Time: Totals:						

Mid-Afternoon Snack	Calories	Protein	Carbs	Fiber	Fat	Added Sugar
Time: Totals:						

Dinner	Calories	Protein	Carbs	Fiber	Fat	Added Sugar
Time: Totals:						

Evening Snack	Calories	Protein	Carbs	Fiber	Fat	Added Sugar
Time: Totals:						

Daily Totals	Calories	Protein	Carbs	Fiber	Fat	Added Sugar
Totals for all Meals and Snacks:						

Fitness Activity   Time   Duration

_____

_____

Daily Food Log　　　　Day:_____　　Date:_____

Hours of Sleep Last Night:　☐ 0-2　　☐ 2-4　　☐ 4-6　　☐ 6-8　　☐ 8-10　　☐ 10+

# of 8 oz. glasses of water consumed:　☐ ☐ ☐ ☐ ☐ ☐ ☐ ☐ ☐ ☐

Vitamins, Supplements, Medications:

Breakfast	Calories	Protein	Carbs	Fiber	Fat	Added Sugar

Time:　　　Totals:

Mid-Morning Snack	Calories	Protein	Carbs	Fiber	Fat	Added Sugar

Time:　　　Totals:

Lunch	Calories	Protein	Carbs	Fiber	Fat	Added Sugar

Time:　　　Totals:

Mid-Afternoon Snack	Calories	Protein	Carbs	Fiber	Fat	Added Sugar
Time: Totals:						

Dinner	Calories	Protein	Carbs	Fiber	Fat	Added Sugar
Time: Totals:						

Evening Snack	Calories	Protein	Carbs	Fiber	Fat	Added Sugar
Time: Totals:						

Daily Totals	Calories	Protein	Carbs	Fiber	Fat	Added Sugar
Totals for all Meals and Snacks:						

Fitness Activity   Time   Duration

_____

_____

Daily Food Log   **Day**:_____   Date:_____

Hours of Sleep Last Night: ☐ 0-2   ☐ 2-4   ☐ 4-6   ☐ 6-8   ☐ 8-10   ☐ 10+

# of 8 oz. glasses of water consumed: ☐ ☐ ☐ ☐ ☐ ☐ ☐ ☐ ☐ ☐

Vitamins, Supplements, Medications:

Breakfast	Calories	Protein	Carbs	Fiber	Fat	Added Sugar
Time: Totals:						

Mid-Morning Snack	Calories	Protein	Carbs	Fiber	Fat	Added Sugar
Time: Totals:						

Lunch	Calories	Protein	Carbs	Fiber	Fat	Added Sugar
Time: Totals:						

Mid-Afternoon Snack	Calories	Protein	Carbs	Fiber	Fat	Added Sugar
Time: Totals:						

Dinner	Calories	Protein	Carbs	Fiber	Fat	Added Sugar
Time: Totals:						

Evening Snack	Calories	Protein	Carbs	Fiber	Fat	Added Sugar
Time: Totals:						

Daily Totals	Calories	Protein	Carbs	Fiber	Fat	Added Sugar
Totals for all Meals and Snacks:						

Fitness Activity   Time   Duration

_____

_____

Daily Food Log   Day:_____   Date:_____

Hours of Sleep Last Night: ☐ 0-2   ☐ 2-4   ☐ 4-6   ☐ 6-8   ☐ 8-10   ☐ 10+

# of 8 oz. glasses of water consumed: ☐ ☐ ☐ ☐ ☐ ☐ ☐ ☐ ☐ ☐

Vitamins, Supplements, Medications:

Breakfast	Calories	Protein	Carbs	Fiber	Fat	Added Sugar
_____						
_____						
_____						
Time: Totals:						

Mid-Morning Snack	Calories	Protein	Carbs	Fiber	Fat	Added Sugar
_____						
_____						
Time: Totals:						

Lunch	Calories	Protein	Carbs	Fiber	Fat	Added Sugar
_____						
_____						
_____						
Time: Totals:						

Mid-Afternoon Snack	Calories	Protein	Carbs	Fiber	Fat	Added Sugar
Time: Totals:						

Dinner	Calories	Protein	Carbs	Fiber	Fat	Added Sugar
Time: Totals:						

Evening Snack	Calories	Protein	Carbs	Fiber	Fat	Added Sugar
Time: Totals:						

Daily Totals	Calories	Protein	Carbs	Fiber	Fat	Added Sugar
Totals for all Meals and Snacks:						

Fitness Activity   Time   Duration

_____

_____

Daily Food Log   Day:_____   Date:_____

Hours of Sleep Last Night: ☐ 0-2   ☐ 2-4   ☐ 4-6   ☐ 6-8   ☐ 8-10   ☐ 10+

# of 8 oz. glasses of water consumed: ☐ ☐ ☐ ☐ ☐ ☐ ☐ ☐ ☐ ☐

Vitamins, Supplements, Medications:

Breakfast	Calories	Protein	Carbs	Fiber	Fat	Added Sugar

Time: Totals:

Mid-Morning Snack	Calories	Protein	Carbs	Fiber	Fat	Added Sugar

Time: Totals:

Lunch	Calories	Protein	Carbs	Fiber	Fat	Added Sugar

Time: Totals:

Mid-Afternoon Snack	Calories	Protein	Carbs	Fiber	Fat	Added Sugar
Time: Totals:						

Dinner	Calories	Protein	Carbs	Fiber	Fat	Added Sugar
Time: Totals:						

Evening Snack	Calories	Protein	Carbs	Fiber	Fat	Added Sugar
Time: Totals:						

Daily Totals	Calories	Protein	Carbs	Fiber	Fat	Added Sugar
Totals for all Meals and Snacks:						

Fitness Activity   Time   Duration

_____

_____

Daily Food Log Day:_____ Date:_____

Hours of Sleep Last Night: ☐ 0-2   ☐ 2-4   ☐ 4-6   ☐ 6-8   ☐ 8-10   ☐ 10+

# of 8 oz. glasses of water consumed: ☐ ☐ ☐ ☐ ☐ ☐ ☐ ☐ ☐ ☐

Vitamins, Supplements, Medications:

Breakfast	Calories	Protein	Carbs	Fiber	Fat	Added Sugar
Time: Totals:						

Mid-Morning Snack	Calories	Protein	Carbs	Fiber	Fat	Added Sugar
Time: Totals:						

Lunch	Calories	Protein	Carbs	Fiber	Fat	Added Sugar
Time: Totals:						

Mid-Afternoon Snack	Calories	Protein	Carbs	Fiber	Fat	Added Sugar
Time: Totals:						

Dinner	Calories	Protein	Carbs	Fiber	Fat	Added Sugar
Time: Totals:						

Evening Snack	Calories	Protein	Carbs	Fiber	Fat	Added Sugar
Time: Totals:						

Daily Totals	Calories	Protein	Carbs	Fiber	Fat	Added Sugar
Totals for all Meals and Snacks:						

Fitness Activity   Time   Duration

_____

_____

Week 1 Wrap Up

Did you meet your goals for the week?   ☐ Yes   ☐ No

What helped you reach your goals or what kept you from reaching your goals:

_____

_____

_____

_____

How do you feel about that?

_____

_____

_____

_____

How do you feel about yourself?

_____

_____

_____

_____

Looking back on this past week, what about yourself are you the most proud?

_____

_____

Week 2 Goals

What are your goals for next week?

_____

_____

_____

_____

_____

*"Success is the sum of small efforts,
repeated day in and day out."*

Robert Collier

Daily Food Log   Day:_____   Date:_____

Hours of Sleep Last Night: ☐ 0-2   ☐ 2-4   ☐ 4-6   ☐ 6-8   ☐ 8-10   ☐ 10+

# of 8 oz. glasses of water consumed: ☐ ☐ ☐ ☐ ☐ ☐ ☐ ☐ ☐ ☐

Vitamins, Supplements, Medications:

Breakfast	Calories	Protein	Carbs	Fiber	Fat	Added Sugar
Time: Totals:						

Mid-Morning Snack	Calories	Protein	Carbs	Fiber	Fat	Added Sugar
Time: Totals:						

Lunch	Calories	Protein	Carbs	Fiber	Fat	Added Sugar
Time: Totals:						

Mid-Afternoon Snack	Calories	Protein	Carbs	Fiber	Fat	Added Sugar
Time: Totals:						

Dinner	Calories	Protein	Carbs	Fiber	Fat	Added Sugar
Time: Totals:						

Evening Snack	Calories	Protein	Carbs	Fiber	Fat	Added Sugar
Time: Totals:						

Daily Totals	Calories	Protein	Carbs	Fiber	Fat	Added Sugar
Totals for all Meals and Snacks:						

Fitness Activity   Time   Duration

_____

_____

Daily Food Log   Day:_____   Date:_____

Hours of Sleep Last Night: ☐ 0-2   ☐ 2-4   ☐ 4-6   ☐ 6-8   ☐ 8-10   ☐ 10+

# of 8 oz. glasses of water consumed: ☐ ☐ ☐ ☐ ☐ ☐ ☐ ☐ ☐ ☐

Vitamins, Supplements, Medications:

Breakfast	Calories	Protein	Carbs	Fiber	Fat	Added Sugar
Time: Totals:						

Mid-Morning Snack	Calories	Protein	Carbs	Fiber	Fat	Added Sugar
Time: Totals:						

Lunch	Calories	Protein	Carbs	Fiber	Fat	Added Sugar
Time: Totals:						

Mid-Afternoon Snack	Calories	Protein	Carbs	Fiber	Fat	Added Sugar
Time: Totals:						

Dinner	Calories	Protein	Carbs	Fiber	Fat	Added Sugar
Time: Totals:						

Evening Snack	Calories	Protein	Carbs	Fiber	Fat	Added Sugar
Time: Totals:						

Daily Totals	Calories	Protein	Carbs	Fiber	Fat	Added Sugar
Totals for all Meals and Snacks:						

Fitness Activity   Time   Duration

_____

_____

Daily Food Log   Day:_____   Date:_____

Hours of Sleep Last Night: ☐ 0-2   ☐ 2-4   ☐ 4-6   ☐ 6-8   ☐ 8-10   ☐ 10+

# of 8 oz. glasses of water consumed: ☐ ☐ ☐ ☐ ☐ ☐ ☐ ☐ ☐ ☐

Vitamins, Supplements, Medications:

Breakfast	Calories	Protein	Carbs	Fiber	Fat	Added Sugar
Time: Totals:						

Mid-Morning Snack	Calories	Protein	Carbs	Fiber	Fat	Added Sugar
Time: Totals:						

Lunch	Calories	Protein	Carbs	Fiber	Fat	Added Sugar
Time: Totals:						

Mid-Afternoon Snack	Calories	Protein	Carbs	Fiber	Fat	Added Sugar
Time: Totals:						

Dinner	Calories	Protein	Carbs	Fiber	Fat	Added Sugar
Time: Totals:						

Evening Snack	Calories	Protein	Carbs	Fiber	Fat	Added Sugar
Time: Totals:						

Daily Totals	Calories	Protein	Carbs	Fiber	Fat	Added Sugar
Totals for all Meals and Snacks:						

Fitness Activity   Time   Duration

_____

_____

Daily Food Log   **Day**:_____   Date:_____

Hours of Sleep Last Night: ☐ 0-2   ☐ 2-4   ☐ 4-6   ☐ 6-8   ☐ 8-10   ☐ 10+

# of 8 oz. glasses of water consumed: ☐ ☐ ☐ ☐ ☐ ☐ ☐ ☐ ☐ ☐

Vitamins, Supplements, Medications:

Breakfast	Calories	Protein	Carbs	Fiber	Fat	Added Sugar
Time: Totals:						

Mid-Morning Snack	Calories	Protein	Carbs	Fiber	Fat	Added Sugar
Time: Totals:						

Lunch	Calories	Protein	Carbs	Fiber	Fat	Added Sugar
Time: Totals:						

Mid-Afternoon Snack	Calories	Protein	Carbs	Fiber	Fat	Added Sugar
Time: Totals:						

Dinner	Calories	Protein	Carbs	Fiber	Fat	Added Sugar
Time: Totals:						

Evening Snack	Calories	Protein	Carbs	Fiber	Fat	Added Sugar
Time: Totals:						

Daily Totals	Calories	Protein	Carbs	Fiber	Fat	Added Sugar
Totals for all Meals and Snacks:						

Fitness Activity   Time   Duration

_____

_____

Daily Food Log   Day:_____   Date:_____

Hours of Sleep Last Night: ☐ 0-2   ☐ 2-4   ☐ 4-6   ☐ 6-8   ☐ 8-10   ☐ 10+

# of 8 oz. glasses of water consumed: ☐ ☐ ☐ ☐ ☐ ☐ ☐ ☐ ☐ ☐

Vitamins, Supplements, Medications:

Breakfast	Calories	Protein	Carbs	Fiber	Fat	Added Sugar
Time: Totals:						

Mid-Morning Snack	Calories	Protein	Carbs	Fiber	Fat	Added Sugar
Time: Totals:						

Lunch	Calories	Protein	Carbs	Fiber	Fat	Added Sugar
Time: Totals:						

Mid-Afternoon Snack	Calories	Protein	Carbs	Fiber	Fat	Added Sugar
Time: Totals:						

Dinner	Calories	Protein	Carbs	Fiber	Fat	Added Sugar
Time: Totals:						

Evening Snack	Calories	Protein	Carbs	Fiber	Fat	Added Sugar
Time: Totals:						

Daily Totals	Calories	Protein	Carbs	Fiber	Fat	Added Sugar
Totals for all Meals and Snacks:						

Fitness Activity   Time   Duration

_____

_____

Daily Food Log   Day:_____   Date:_____

Hours of Sleep Last Night: ☐ 0-2   ☐ 2-4   ☐ 4-6   ☐ 6-8   ☐ 8-10   ☐ 10+

# of 8 oz. glasses of water consumed: ☐ ☐ ☐ ☐ ☐ ☐ ☐ ☐ ☐ ☐

Vitamins, Supplements, Medications:

Breakfast	Calories	Protein	Carbs	Fiber	Fat	Added Sugar
Time: Totals:						

Mid-Morning Snack	Calories	Protein	Carbs	Fiber	Fat	Added Sugar
Time: Totals:						

Lunch	Calories	Protein	Carbs	Fiber	Fat	Added Sugar
Time: Totals:						Added

Mid-Afternoon Snack	Calories	Protein	Carbs	Fiber	Fat	Sugar
Time: Totals:						

Dinner	Calories	Protein	Carbs	Fiber	Fat	Added Sugar
Time: Totals:						

Evening Snack	Calories	Protein	Carbs	Fiber	Fat	Added Sugar
Time: Totals:						

Daily Totals	Calories	Protein	Carbs	Fiber	Fat	Added Sugar
Totals for all Meals and Snacks:						

Fitness Activity   Time   Duration

_____

_____

Daily Food Log Day:_____ Date:_____

Hours of Sleep Last Night: ☐ 0-2 ☐ 2-4 ☐ 4-6 ☐ 6-8 ☐ 8-10 ☐ 10+

# of 8 oz. glasses of water consumed: ☐ ☐ ☐ ☐ ☐ ☐ ☐ ☐ ☐ ☐

Vitamins, Supplements, Medications:

Breakfast	Calories	Protein	Carbs	Fiber	Fat	Added Sugar
Time: Totals:						

Mid-Morning Snack	Calories	Protein	Carbs	Fiber	Fat	Added Sugar
Time: Totals:						

Lunch	Calories	Protein	Carbs	Fiber	Fat	Added Sugar
Time: Totals:						

Mid-Afternoon Snack	Calories	Protein	Carbs	Fiber	Fat	Added Sugar
Time: Totals:						

Dinner	Calories	Protein	Carbs	Fiber	Fat	Added Sugar
Time: Totals:						

Evening Snack	Calories	Protein	Carbs	Fiber	Fat	Added Sugar
Time: Totals:						

Daily Totals	Calories	Protein	Carbs	Fiber	Fat	Added Sugar
Totals for all Meals and Snacks:						

Fitness Activity   Time   Duration

_____

_____

Week 2 Wrap Up

Did you meet your goals for the week?   ☐ Yes   ☐ No

What helped you reach your goals or what kept you from reaching your goals:

_____

_____

_____

_____

How do you feel about that?

_____

_____

_____

_____

How do you feel about yourself?

_____

_____

_____

_____

Looking back on this past week, what about yourself are you the most proud?

_____

_____

Week 3 Goals

What are your goals for next week?

_____

_____

_____

_____

_____

*"You must expect great things of yourself
before you can do them."*

Michael Jordan

Daily Food Log Day:_____ Date:_____

Hours of Sleep Last Night: ☐ 0-2   ☐ 2-4   ☐ 4-6   ☐ 6-8   ☐ 8-10   ☐ 10+

# of 8 oz. glasses of water consumed: ☐ ☐ ☐ ☐ ☐ ☐ ☐ ☐ ☐ ☐

Vitamins, Supplements, Medications::

Breakfast	Calories	Protein	Carbs	Fiber	Fat	Added Sugar

Time: Totals:

Mid-Morning Snack	Calories	Protein	Carbs	Fiber	Fat	Added Sugar

Time: Totals:

Lunch	Calories	Protein	Carbs	Fiber	Fat	Added Sugar

Time: Totals:

Mid-Afternoon Snack	Calories	Protein	Carbs	Fiber	Fat	Added Sugar
Time: Totals:						

Dinner	Calories	Protein	Carbs	Fiber	Fat	Added Sugar
Time: Totals:						

Evening Snack	Calories	Protein	Carbs	Fiber	Fat	Added Sugar
Time: Totals:						

Daily Totals	Calories	Protein	Carbs	Fiber	Fat	Added Sugar
Totals for all Meals and Snacks:						

Fitness Activity   Time   Duration

_____

_____

Daily Food Log　　　　　Day:_____　　　Date:_____

Hours of Sleep Last Night:　☐ 0-2　　☐ 2-4　　☐ 4-6　　☐ 6-8　　☐ 8-10　　☐ 10+

# of 8 oz. glasses of water consumed: ☐ ☐ ☐ ☐ ☐ ☐ ☐ ☐ ☐ ☐

Vitamins, Supplements, Medications:

Breakfast	Calories	Protein	Carbs	Fiber	Fat	Added Sugar
Time:　　　Totals:						

Mid-Morning Snack	Calories	Protein	Carbs	Fiber	Fat	Added Sugar
Time:　　　Totals:						

Lunch	Calories	Protein	Carbs	Fiber	Fat	Added Sugar
Time:　　　Totals:						

Mid-Afternoon Snack	Calories	Protein	Carbs	Fiber	Fat	Added Sugar
Time: Totals:						

Dinner	Calories	Protein	Carbs	Fiber	Fat	Added Sugar
Time: Totals:						

Evening Snack	Calories	Protein	Carbs	Fiber	Fat	Added Sugar
Time: Totals:						

Daily Totals	Calories	Protein	Carbs	Fiber	Fat	Added Sugar
Totals for all Meals and Snacks:						

Fitness Activity   Time   Duration

_____

_____

Daily Food Log   Day:_____   Date:_____

Hours of Sleep Last Night: ☐ 0-2   ☐ 2-4   ☐ 4-6   ☐ 6-8   ☐ 8-10   ☐ 10+

# of 8 oz. glasses of water consumed: ☐ ☐ ☐ ☐ ☐ ☐ ☐ ☐ ☐ ☐

Vitamins, Supplements, Medications:

Breakfast	Calories	Protein	Carbs	Fiber	Fat	Added Sugar

Time: Totals:

Mid-Morning Snack	Calories	Protein	Carbs	Fiber	Fat	Added Sugar

Time: Totals:

Lunch	Calories	Protein	Carbs	Fiber	Fat	Added Sugar

Time: Totals:

Mid-Afternoon Snack	Calories	Protein	Carbs	Fiber	Fat	Added Sugar
Time: Totals:						

Dinner	Calories	Protein	Carbs	Fiber	Fat	Added Sugar
Time: Totals:						

Evening Snack	Calories	Protein	Carbs	Fiber	Fat	Added Sugar
Time: Totals:						

Daily Totals	Calories	Protein	Carbs	Fiber	Fat	Added Sugar
Totals for all Meals and Snacks:						

Fitness Activity   Time   Duration

_____

_____

Daily Food Log   **Day**:_____   Date:_____

Hours of Sleep Last Night: ☐ 0-2   ☐ 2-4   ☐ 4-6   ☐ 6-8   ☐ 8-10   ☐ 10+

# of 8 oz. glasses of water consumed: ☐ ☐ ☐ ☐ ☐ ☐ ☐ ☐ ☐ ☐

Vitamins, Supplements, Medications:

Breakfast	Calories	Protein	Carbs	Fiber	Fat	Added Sugar

Time: Totals:

Mid-Morning Snack	Calories	Protein	Carbs	Fiber	Fat	Added Sugar

Time: Totals:

Lunch	Calories	Protein	Carbs	Fiber	Fat	Added Sugar

Time: Totals:

Mid-Afternoon Snack	Calories	Protein	Carbs	Fiber	Fat	Added Sugar
Time: Totals:						

Dinner	Calories	Protein	Carbs	Fiber	Fat	Added Sugar
Time: Totals:						

Evening Snack	Calories	Protein	Carbs	Fiber	Fat	Added Sugar
Time: Totals:						

Daily Totals	Calories	Protein	Carbs	Fiber	Fat	Added Sugar
Totals for all Meals and Snacks:						

Fitness Activity   Time   Duration

_____

_____

Daily Food Log   Day:_____   Date:_____

Hours of Sleep Last Night: ☐ 0-2   ☐ 2-4   ☐ 4-6   ☐ 6-8   ☐ 8-10   ☐ 10+

# of 8 oz. glasses of water consumed: ☐ ☐ ☐ ☐ ☐ ☐ ☐ ☐ ☐ ☐

Vitamins, Supplements, Medications:

Breakfast	Calories	Protein	Carbs	Fiber	Fat	Added Sugar

Time: Totals:

Mid-Morning Snack	Calories	Protein	Carbs	Fiber	Fat	Added Sugar

Time: Totals:

Lunch	Calories	Protein	Carbs	Fiber	Fat	Added Sugar

Time: Totals:

Mid-Afternoon Snack	Calories	Protein	Carbs	Fiber	Fat	Added Sugar
Time: Totals:						

Dinner	Calories	Protein	Carbs	Fiber	Fat	Added Sugar
Time: Totals:						

Evening Snack	Calories	Protein	Carbs	Fiber	Fat	Added Sugar
Time: Totals:						

Daily Totals	Calories	Protein	Carbs	Fiber	Fat	Added Sugar
Totals for all Meals and Snacks:						

Fitness Activity   Time   Duration

_____

_____

Daily Food Log   Day:_____   Date:_____

Hours of Sleep Last Night: ☐ 0-2   ☐ 2-4   ☐ 4-6   ☐ 6-8   ☐ 8-10   ☐ 10+

# of 8 oz. glasses of water consumed: ☐ ☐ ☐ ☐ ☐ ☐ ☐ ☐ ☐ ☐

Vitamins, Supplements, Medications:

Breakfast	Calories	Protein	Carbs	Fiber	Fat	Added Sugar

Time: Totals:

Mid-Morning Snack	Calories	Protein	Carbs	Fiber	Fat	Added Sugar

Time: Totals:

Lunch	Calories	Protein	Carbs	Fiber	Fat	Added Sugar

Time: Totals:

Mid-Afternoon Snack	Calories	Protein	Carbs	Fiber	Fat	Added Sugar
Time: Totals:						

Dinner	Calories	Protein	Carbs	Fiber	Fat	Added Sugar
Time: Totals:						

Evening Snack	Calories	Protein	Carbs	Fiber	Fat	Added Sugar
Time: Totals:						

Daily Totals	Calories	Protein	Carbs	Fiber	Fat	Added Sugar
Totals for all Meals and Snacks:						

Fitness Activity   Time   Duration

_____

_____

Daily Food Log   Day:_____   Date:_____

Hours of Sleep Last Night: ☐ 0-2   ☐ 2-4   ☐ 4-6   ☐ 6-8   ☐ 8-10   ☐ 10+

# of 8 oz. glasses of water consumed: ☐ ☐ ☐ ☐ ☐ ☐ ☐ ☐ ☐ ☐

Vitamins, Supplements, Medications:

Breakfast	Calories	Protein	Carbs	Fiber	Fat	Added Sugar
Time: Totals:						

Mid-Morning Snack	Calories	Protein	Carbs	Fiber	Fat	Added Sugar
Time: Totals:						

Lunch	Calories	Protein	Carbs	Fiber	Fat	Added Sugar
Time: Totals:						

Mid-Afternoon Snack	Calories	Protein	Carbs	Fiber	Fat	Added Sugar
Time: Totals:						

Dinner	Calories	Protein	Carbs	Fiber	Fat	Added Sugar
Time: Totals:						

Evening Snack	Calories	Protein	Carbs	Fiber	Fat	Added Sugar
Time: Totals:						

Daily Totals	Calories	Protein	Carbs	Fiber	Fat	Added Sugar
Totals for all Meals and Snacks:						

Fitness Activity   Time   Duration

_____

_____

Week 3 Wrap Up

Did you meet your goals for the week?   ☐ Yes   ☐ No

What helped you reach your goals or what kept you from reaching your goals:

_____

_____

_____

_____

How do you feel about that?

_____

_____

_____

_____

How do you feel about yourself?

_____

_____

_____

_____

Looking back on this past week, what about yourself are you the most proud?

_____

_____

Week 4 Goals

What are your goals for next week?

_____

_____

_____

_____

_____

"We've got to remember that we get whatever we focus on in life. If we keep focusing on what we don't want, we'll have more of it. The first step to creating any change is deciding what you do want so that you have something to move toward."

Anthony Robbins

Daily Food Log   Day:_____   Date:_____

Hours of Sleep Last Night: ☐ 0-2   ☐ 2-4   ☐ 4-6   ☐ 6-8   ☐ 8-10   ☐ 10+

# of 8 oz. glasses of water consumed: ☐ ☐ ☐ ☐ ☐ ☐ ☐ ☐ ☐ ☐

Vitamins, Supplements, Medications:

Breakfast	Calories	Protein	Carbs	Fiber	Fat	Added Sugar

Time: Totals:

Mid-Morning Snack	Calories	Protein	Carbs	Fiber	Fat	Added Sugar

Time: Totals:

Lunch	Calories	Protein	Carbs	Fiber	Fat	Added Sugar

Time: Totals:

Mid-Afternoon Snack	Calories	Protein	Carbs	Fiber	Fat	Added Sugar
Time: Totals:						

Dinner	Calories	Protein	Carbs	Fiber	Fat	Added Sugar
Time: Totals:						

Evening Snack	Calories	Protein	Carbs	Fiber	Fat	Added Sugar
Time: Totals:						

Daily Totals	Calories	Protein	Carbs	Fiber	Fat	Added Sugar
Totals for all Meals and Snacks:						

Fitness Activity   Time   Duration

_____

_____

Daily Food Log   Day:_____   Date:_____

Hours of Sleep Last Night: ☐ 0-2   ☐ 2-4   ☐ 4-6   ☐ 6-8   ☐ 8-10   ☐ 10+

# of 8 oz. glasses of water consumed: ☐ ☐ ☐ ☐ ☐ ☐ ☐ ☐ ☐ ☐

Vitamins, Supplements, Medications:

Breakfast	Calories	Protein	Carbs	Fiber	Fat	Added Sugar

Time: Totals:

Mid-Morning Snack	Calories	Protein	Carbs	Fiber	Fat	Added Sugar

Time: Totals:

Lunch	Calories	Protein	Carbs	Fiber	Fat	Added Sugar

Time: Totals:

Mid-Afternoon Snack	Calories	Protein	Carbs	Fiber	Fat	Added Sugar
Time: Totals:						

Dinner	Calories	Protein	Carbs	Fiber	Fat	Added Sugar
Time: Totals:						

Evening Snack	Calories	Protein	Carbs	Fiber	Fat	Added Sugar
Time: Totals:						

Daily Totals	Calories	Protein	Carbs	Fiber	Fat	Added Sugar
Totals for all Meals and Snacks:						

Fitness Activity   Time   Duration

_____

_____

Daily Food Log   Day:_____   Date:_____

Hours of Sleep Last Night: ☐ 0-2   ☐ 2-4   ☐ 4-6   ☐ 6-8   ☐ 8-10   ☐ 10+

# of 8 oz. glasses of water consumed: ☐ ☐ ☐ ☐ ☐ ☐ ☐ ☐ ☐

Vitamins, Supplements, Medications:

Breakfast	Calories	Protein	Carbs	Fiber	Fat	Added Sugar

Time: Totals:

Mid-Morning Snack	Calories	Protein	Carbs	Fiber	Fat	Added Sugar

Time: Totals:

Lunch	Calories	Protein	Carbs	Fiber	Fat	Added Sugar

Time: Totals:

Mid-Afternoon Snack	Calories	Protein	Carbs	Fiber	Fat	Added Sugar
Time: Totals:						

Dinner	Calories	Protein	Carbs	Fiber	Fat	Added Sugar
Time: Totals:						

Evening Snack	Calories	Protein	Carbs	Fiber	Fat	Added Sugar
Time: Totals:						

Daily Totals	Calories	Protein	Carbs	Fiber	Fat	Added Sugar
Totals for all Meals and Snacks:						

Fitness Activity Time Duration

_____

_____

Daily Food Log   **Day**:_____   Date:_____

Hours of Sleep Last Night: ☐ 0-2   ☐ 2-4   ☐ 4-6   ☐ 6-8   ☐ 8-10   ☐ 10+

# of 8 oz. glasses of water consumed: ☐ ☐ ☐ ☐ ☐ ☐ ☐ ☐ ☐ ☐

Vitamins, Supplements, Medications:

Breakfast	Calories	Protein	Carbs	Fiber	Fat	Added Sugar
Time: Totals:						

Mid-Morning Snack	Calories	Protein	Carbs	Fiber	Fat	Added Sugar
Time: Totals:						

Lunch	Calories	Protein	Carbs	Fiber	Fat	Added Sugar
Time: Totals:						

Mid-Afternoon Snack	Calories	Protein	Carbs	Fiber	Fat	Added Sugar
Time: Totals:						

Dinner	Calories	Protein	Carbs	Fiber	Fat	Added Sugar
Time: Totals:						

Evening Snack	Calories	Protein	Carbs	Fiber	Fat	Added Sugar
Time: Totals:						

Daily Totals	Calories	Protein	Carbs	Fiber	Fat	Added Sugar
Totals for all Meals and Snacks:						

Fitness Activity   Time   Duration

_____

_____

Daily Food Log   Day:_____   Date:_____

Hours of Sleep Last Night: ☐ 0-2   ☐ 2-4   ☐ 4-6   ☐ 6-8   ☐ 8-10   ☐ 10+

# of 8 oz. glasses of water consumed: ☐ ☐ ☐ ☐ ☐ ☐ ☐ ☐ ☐ ☐

Vitamins, Supplements, Medications:

Breakfast	Calories	Protein	Carbs	Fiber	Fat	Added Sugar

Time: Totals:

Mid-Morning Snack	Calories	Protein	Carbs	Fiber	Fat	Added Sugar

Time: Totals:

Lunch	Calories	Protein	Carbs	Fiber	Fat	Added Sugar

Time: Totals:

Mid-Afternoon Snack	Calories	Protein	Carbs	Fiber	Fat	Added Sugar
Time: Totals:						

Dinner	Calories	Protein	Carbs	Fiber	Fat	Added Sugar
Time: Totals:						

Evening Snack	Calories	Protein	Carbs	Fiber	Fat	Added Sugar
Time: Totals:						

Daily Totals	Calories	Protein	Carbs	Fiber	Fat	Added Sugar
Totals for all Meals and Snacks:						

Fitness Activity   Time   Duration

_____

_____

Daily Food Log   Day:_____   Date:_____

Hours of Sleep Last Night: ☐ 0-2   ☐ 2-4   ☐ 4-6   ☐ 6-8   ☐ 8-10   ☐ 10+

# of 8 oz. glasses of water consumed: ☐ ☐ ☐ ☐ ☐ ☐ ☐ ☐ ☐ ☐

Vitamins, Supplements, Medications:

Breakfast	Calories	Protein	Carbs	Fiber	Fat	Added Sugar
Time: Totals:						

Mid-Morning Snack	Calories	Protein	Carbs	Fiber	Fat	Added Sugar
Time: Totals:						

Lunch	Calories	Protein	Carbs	Fiber	Fat	Added Sugar
Time: Totals:						

Mid-Afternoon Snack	Calories	Protein	Carbs	Fiber	Fat	Added Sugar
Time: Totals:						

Dinner	Calories	Protein	Carbs	Fiber	Fat	Added Sugar
Time: Totals:						

Evening Snack	Calories	Protein	Carbs	Fiber	Fat	Added Sugar
Time: Totals:						

Daily Totals	Calories	Protein	Carbs	Fiber	Fat	Added Sugar
Totals for all Meals and Snacks:						

Fitness Activity   Time   Duration

_____

_____

Daily Food Log Day:_____ Date:_____

Hours of Sleep Last Night: ☐ 0-2   ☐ 2-4   ☐ 4-6   ☐ 6-8   ☐ 8-10   ☐ 10+

# of 8 oz. glasses of water consumed: ☐ ☐ ☐ ☐ ☐ ☐ ☐ ☐ ☐ ☐

Vitamins, Supplements, Medications:

Breakfast	Calories	Protein	Carbs	Fiber	Fat	Added Sugar

Time: Totals:

Mid-Morning Snack	Calories	Protein	Carbs	Fiber	Fat	Added Sugar

Time: Totals:

Lunch	Calories	Protein	Carbs	Fiber	Fat	Added Sugar

Time: Totals:

Mid-Afternoon Snack	Calories	Protein	Carbs	Fiber	Fat	Added Sugar
Time: Totals:						

Dinner	Calories	Protein	Carbs	Fiber	Fat	Added Sugar
Time: Totals:						

Evening Snack	Calories	Protein	Carbs	Fiber	Fat	Added Sugar
Time: Totals:						

Daily Totals	Calories	Protein	Carbs	Fiber	Fat	Added Sugar
Totals for all Meals and Snacks:						

Fitness Activity   Time   Duration

_____

_____

Week 4 Wrap Up

Did you meet your goals for the week?   ☐ Yes   ☐ No

What helped you reach your goals or what kept you from reaching your goals:

_____

_____

_____

_____

How do you feel about that?

_____

_____

_____

_____

How do you feel about yourself?

_____

_____

_____

_____

Looking back on this past week, what about yourself are you the most proud?

_____

_____

Week 5 Goals

What are your goals for next week?

_____

_____

_____

_____

_____

"When you have a great and difficult task, something perhaps almost impossible, if you only work a little at a time, every day a little, suddenly the work will finish itself."

Isak Dinesen

Daily Food Log Day:_____ Date:_____

Hours of Sleep Last Night: ☐ 0-2   ☐ 2-4   ☐ 4-6   ☐ 6-8   ☐ 8-10   ☐ 10+

# of 8 oz. glasses of water consumed: ☐ ☐ ☐ ☐ ☐ ☐ ☐ ☐ ☐ ☐

Vitamins, Supplements, Medications:

Breakfast	Calories	Protein	Carbs	Fiber	Fat	Added Sugar
Time: Totals:						

Mid-Morning Snack	Calories	Protein	Carbs	Fiber	Fat	Added Sugar
Time: Totals:						

Lunch	Calories	Protein	Carbs	Fiber	Fat	Added Sugar
Time: Totals:						

Mid-Afternoon Snack	Calories	Protein	Carbs	Fiber	Fat	Added Sugar
Time: Totals:						

Dinner	Calories	Protein	Carbs	Fiber	Fat	Added Sugar
Time: Totals:						

Evening Snack	Calories	Protein	Carbs	Fiber	Fat	Added Sugar
Time: Totals:						

Daily Totals	Calories	Protein	Carbs	Fiber	Fat	Added Sugar
Totals for all Meals and Snacks:						

Fitness Activity   Time   Duration

_____

_____

Daily Food Log   Day:_____   Date:_____

Hours of Sleep Last Night: ☐ 0-2   ☐ 2-4   ☐ 4-6   ☐ 6-8   ☐ 8-10   ☐ 10+

# of 8 oz. glasses of water consumed: ☐ ☐ ☐ ☐ ☐ ☐ ☐ ☐ ☐ ☐

Vitamins, Supplements, Medications:

Breakfast	Calories	Protein	Carbs	Fiber	Fat	Added Sugar
Time: Totals:						

Mid-Morning Snack	Calories	Protein	Carbs	Fiber	Fat	Added Sugar
Time: Totals:						

Lunch	Calories	Protein	Carbs	Fiber	Fat	Added Sugar
Time: Totals:						

Mid-Afternoon Snack	Calories	Protein	Carbs	Fiber	Fat	Added Sugar
Time: Totals:						

Dinner	Calories	Protein	Carbs	Fiber	Fat	Added Sugar
Time: Totals:						

Evening Snack	Calories	Protein	Carbs	Fiber	Fat	Added Sugar
Time: Totals:						

Daily Totals	Calories	Protein	Carbs	Fiber	Fat	Added Sugar
Totals for all Meals and Snacks:						

Fitness Activity   Time   Duration
_____

_____

Daily Food Log Day:_____ Date:_____

Hours of Sleep Last Night: ☐ 0-2 ☐ 2-4 ☐ 4-6 ☐ 6-8 ☐ 8-10 ☐ 10+

# of 8 oz. glasses of water consumed: ☐ ☐ ☐ ☐ ☐ ☐ ☐ ☐ ☐

Vitamins, Supplements, Medications:

Breakfast	Calories	Protein	Carbs	Fiber	Fat	Added Sugar
Time: Totals:						

Mid-Morning Snack	Calories	Protein	Carbs	Fiber	Fat	Added Sugar
Time: Totals:						

Lunch	Calories	Protein	Carbs	Fiber	Fat	Added Sugar
Time: Totals:						

Mid-Afternoon Snack	Calories	Protein	Carbs	Fiber	Fat	Added Sugar

Time: Totals:

Dinner	Calories	Protein	Carbs	Fiber	Fat	Added Sugar

Time: Totals:

Evening Snack	Calories	Protein	Carbs	Fiber	Fat	Added Sugar

Time: Totals:

Daily Totals	Calories	Protein	Carbs	Fiber	Fat	Added Sugar
Totals for all Meals and Snacks:						

Fitness Activity   Time   Duration

Daily Food Log   Day:_____   Date:_____

Hours of Sleep Last Night: ☐ 0-2   ☐ 2-4   ☐ 4-6   ☐ 6-8   ☐ 8-10   ☐ 10+

# of 8 oz. glasses of water consumed: ☐ ☐ ☐ ☐ ☐ ☐ ☐ ☐ ☐

Vitamins, Supplements, Medications:

Breakfast	Calories	Protein	Carbs	Fiber	Fat	Added Sugar
Time: Totals:						

Mid-Morning Snack	Calories	Protein	Carbs	Fiber	Fat	Added Sugar
Time: Totals:						

Lunch	Calories	Protein	Carbs	Fiber	Fat	Added Sugar
Time: Totals:						

Mid-Afternoon Snack	Calories	Protein	Carbs	Fiber	Fat	Added Sugar
Time: Totals:						

Dinner	Calories	Protein	Carbs	Fiber	Fat	Added Sugar
Time: Totals:						

Evening Snack	Calories	Protein	Carbs	Fiber	Fat	Added Sugar
Time: Totals:						

Daily Totals	Calories	Protein	Carbs	Fiber	Fat	Added Sugar
Totals for all Meals and Snacks:						

Fitness Activity _____   Time   Duration

_____

_____

Daily Food Log Day:_____ Date:_____

Hours of Sleep Last Night: ☐ 0-2 ☐ 2-4 ☐ 4-6 ☐ 6-8 ☐ 8-10 ☐ 10+

# of 8 oz. glasses of water consumed: ☐ ☐ ☐ ☐ ☐ ☐ ☐ ☐ ☐ ☐

Vitamins, Supplements, Medications:

Breakfast	Calories	Protein	Carbs	Fiber	Fat	Added Sugar
Time: Totals:						

Mid-Morning Snack	Calories	Protein	Carbs	Fiber	Fat	Added Sugar
Time: Totals:						

Lunch	Calories	Protein	Carbs	Fiber	Fat	Added Sugar
Time: Totals:						

Mid-Afternoon Snack	Calories	Protein	Carbs	Fiber	Fat	Added Sugar
Time: Totals:						

Dinner	Calories	Protein	Carbs	Fiber	Fat	Added Sugar
Time: Totals:						

Evening Snack	Calories	Protein	Carbs	Fiber	Fat	Added Sugar
Time: Totals:						

Daily Totals	Calories	Protein	Carbs	Fiber	Fat	Added Sugar
Totals for all Meals and Snacks:						

Fitness Activity   Time   Duration

_____

_____

Daily Food Log

Day:_____   Date:_____

Hours of Sleep Last Night: ☐ 0-2 ☐ 2-4 ☐ 4-6 ☐ 6-8 ☐ 8-10 ☐ 10+

# of 8 oz. glasses of water consumed: ☐ ☐ ☐ ☐ ☐ ☐ ☐ ☐ ☐ ☐

Vitamins, Supplements, Medications:

Breakfast

	Calories	Protein	Carbs	Fiber	Fat	Added Sugar

Time: _____   Totals:

Mid-Morning Snack

	Calories	Protein	Carbs	Fiber	Fat	Added Sugar

Time: _____   Totals:

Lunch

	Calories	Protein	Carbs	Fiber	Fat	Added Sugar

Time: _____   Totals:

Mid-Afternoon Snack	Calories	Protein	Carbs	Fiber	Fat	Added Sugar
Time: Totals:						

Dinner	Calories	Protein	Carbs	Fiber	Fat	Added Sugar
Time: Totals:						

Evening Snack	Calories	Protein	Carbs	Fiber	Fat	Added Sugar
Time: Totals:						

Daily Totals	Calories	Protein	Carbs	Fiber	Fat	Added Sugar
Totals for all Meals and Snacks:						

Fitness Activity   Time   Duration

_____

_____

Daily Food Log   Day:_____   Date:_____

Hours of Sleep Last Night: ☐ 0-2   ☐ 2-4   ☐ 4-6   ☐ 6-8   ☐ 8-10   ☐ 10+

# of 8 oz. glasses of water consumed: ☐ ☐ ☐ ☐ ☐ ☐ ☐ ☐ ☐

Vitamins, Supplements, Medications:

Breakfast	Calories	Protein	Carbs	Fiber	Fat	Added Sugar
Time: Totals:						

Mid-Morning Snack	Calories	Protein	Carbs	Fiber	Fat	Added Sugar
Time: Totals:						

Lunch	Calories	Protein	Carbs	Fiber	Fat	Added Sugar
Time: Totals:						

Mid-Afternoon Snack	Calories	Protein	Carbs	Fiber	Fat	Added Sugar
Time: Totals:						

Dinner	Calories	Protein	Carbs	Fiber	Fat	Added Sugar
Time: Totals:						

Evening Snack	Calories	Protein	Carbs	Fiber	Fat	Added Sugar
Time: Totals:						

Daily Totals	Calories	Protein	Carbs	Fiber	Fat	Added Sugar
Totals for all Meals and Snacks:						

Fitness Activity   Time   Duration

Week 5 Wrap Up

Did you meet your goals for the week?   ☐ Yes   ☐ No

What helped you reach your goals or what kept you from reaching your goals:

_____

_____

_____

_____

How do you feel about that?

_____

_____

_____

_____

How do you feel about yourself?

_____

_____

_____

_____

Looking back on this past week, what about yourself are you the most proud?

_____

_____

Week 6 Goals

What are your goals for next week?

_____

_____

_____

_____

_____

"You aren't going to find anybody that's going to be successful without making a sacrifice and without perseverance."

Lou Holtz

Daily Food Log   Day:_____   Date:_____

Hours of Sleep Last Night: ☐ 0-2   ☐ 2-4   ☐ 4-6   ☐ 6-8   ☐ 8-10   ☐ 10+

# of 8 oz. glasses of water consumed: ☐ ☐ ☐ ☐ ☐ ☐ ☐ ☐ ☐

Vitamins, Supplements, Medications:

Breakfast	Calories	Protein	Carbs	Fiber	Fat	Added Sugar
Time: Totals:						

Mid-Morning Snack	Calories	Protein	Carbs	Fiber	Fat	Added Sugar
Time: Totals:						

Lunch	Calories	Protein	Carbs	Fiber	Fat	Added Sugar
Time: Totals:						

Mid-Afternoon Snack	Calories	Protein	Carbs	Fiber	Fat	Added Sugar
Time: Totals:						

Dinner	Calories	Protein	Carbs	Fiber	Fat	Added Sugar
Time: Totals:						

Evening Snack	Calories	Protein	Carbs	Fiber	Fat	Added Sugar
Time: Totals:						

Daily Totals	Calories	Protein	Carbs	Fiber	Fat	Added Sugar
Totals for all Meals and Snacks:						

Fitness Activity   Time   Duration

_____

_____

Daily Food Log　　　　Day:_____　　　Date:_____

Hours of Sleep Last Night:　☐ 0-2　　☐ 2-4　　☐ 4-6　　☐ 6-8　　☐ 8-10　　☐ 10+

# of 8 oz. glasses of water consumed:　☐ ☐ ☐ ☐ ☐ ☐ ☐ ☐ ☐ ☐

Vitamins, Supplements, Medications:

Breakfast	Calories	Protein	Carbs	Fiber	Fat	Added Sugar
Time:　　　Totals:						

Mid-Morning Snack	Calories	Protein	Carbs	Fiber	Fat	Added Sugar
Time:　　　Totals:						

Lunch	Calories	Protein	Carbs	Fiber	Fat	Added Sugar
Time:　　　Totals:						

Mid-Afternoon Snack	Calories	Protein	Carbs	Fiber	Fat	Added Sugar
Time: Totals:						

Dinner	Calories	Protein	Carbs	Fiber	Fat	Added Sugar
Time: Totals:						

Evening Snack	Calories	Protein	Carbs	Fiber	Fat	Added Sugar
Time: Totals:						

Daily Totals	Calories	Protein	Carbs	Fiber	Fat	Added Sugar
Totals for all Meals and Snacks:						

Fitness Activity   Time   Duration

_____

_____

Daily Food Log   Day:_____   Date:_____

Hours of Sleep Last Night: ☐ 0-2   ☐ 2-4   ☐ 4-6   ☐ 6-8   ☐ 8-10   ☐ 10+

# of 8 oz. glasses of water consumed: ☐ ☐ ☐ ☐ ☐ ☐ ☐ ☐ ☐ ☐

Vitamins, Supplements, Medications:

Breakfast	Calories	Protein	Carbs	Fiber	Fat	Added Sugar
Time: Totals:						

Mid-Morning Snack	Calories	Protein	Carbs	Fiber	Fat	Added Sugar
Time: Totals:						

Lunch	Calories	Protein	Carbs	Fiber	Fat	Added Sugar
Time: Totals:						

Mid-Afternoon Snack	Calories	Protein	Carbs	Fiber	Fat	Added Sugar
Time: Totals:						

Dinner	Calories	Protein	Carbs	Fiber	Fat	Added Sugar
Time: Totals:						

Evening Snack	Calories	Protein	Carbs	Fiber	Fat	Added Sugar
Time: Totals:						

Daily Totals	Calories	Protein	Carbs	Fiber	Fat	Added Sugar
Totals for all Meals and Snacks:						

Fitness Activity   Time   Duration

_____

_____

Daily Food Log   Day:_____   Date:_____

Hours of Sleep Last Night: ☐ 0-2   ☐ 2-4   ☐ 4-6   ☐ 6-8   ☐ 8-10   ☐ 10+

# of 8 oz. glasses of water consumed: ☐ ☐ ☐ ☐ ☐ ☐ ☐ ☐ ☐ ☐

Vitamins, Supplements, Medications:

Breakfast	Calories	Protein	Carbs	Fiber	Fat	Added Sugar

Time: Totals:

Mid-Morning Snack	Calories	Protein	Carbs	Fiber	Fat	Added Sugar

Time: Totals:

Lunch	Calories	Protein	Carbs	Fiber	Fat	Added Sugar

Time: Totals:

Mid-Afternoon Snack	Calories	Protein	Carbs	Fiber	Fat	Added Sugar
Time: Totals:						

Dinner	Calories	Protein	Carbs	Fiber	Fat	Added Sugar
Time: Totals:						

Evening Snack	Calories	Protein	Carbs	Fiber	Fat	Added Sugar
Time: Totals:						

Daily Totals	Calories	Protein	Carbs	Fiber	Fat	Added Sugar
Totals for all Meals and Snacks:						

Fitness Activity   Time   Duration

_____

_____

Daily Food Log   Day:_____   Date:_____

Hours of Sleep Last Night: ☐ 0-2   ☐ 2-4   ☐ 4-6   ☐ 6-8   ☐ 8-10   ☐ 10+

# of 8 oz. glasses of water consumed: ☐ ☐ ☐ ☐ ☐ ☐ ☐ ☐ ☐

Vitamins, Supplements, Medications:

Breakfast	Calories	Protein	Carbs	Fiber	Fat	Added Sugar
Time: Totals:						

Mid-Morning Snack	Calories	Protein	Carbs	Fiber	Fat	Added Sugar
Time: Totals:						

Lunch	Calories	Protein	Carbs	Fiber	Fat	Added Sugar
Time: Totals:						

Mid-Afternoon Snack	Calories	Protein	Carbs	Fiber	Fat	Added Sugar
Time: Totals:						

Dinner	Calories	Protein	Carbs	Fiber	Fat	Added Sugar
Time: Totals:						

Evening Snack	Calories	Protein	Carbs	Fiber	Fat	Added Sugar
Time: Totals:						

Daily Totals	Calories	Protein	Carbs	Fiber	Fat	Added Sugar
Totals for all Meals and Snacks:						

Fitness Activity   Time   Duration

_____

_____

Daily Food Log Day:_____ Date:_____

Hours of Sleep Last Night: ☐ 0-2   ☐ 2-4   ☐ 4-6   ☐ 6-8   ☐ 8-10   ☐ 10+

# of 8 oz. glasses of water consumed: ☐ ☐ ☐ ☐ ☐ ☐ ☐ ☐ ☐

Vitamins, Supplements, Medications:

Breakfast	Calories	Protein	Carbs	Fiber	Fat	Added Sugar
Time: Totals:						

Mid-Morning Snack	Calories	Protein	Carbs	Fiber	Fat	Added Sugar
Time: Totals:						

Lunch	Calories	Protein	Carbs	Fiber	Fat	Added Sugar
Time: Totals:						

Mid-Afternoon Snack	Calories	Protein	Carbs	Fiber	Fat	Added Sugar
Time: Totals:						

Dinner	Calories	Protein	Carbs	Fiber	Fat	Added Sugar
Time: Totals:						

Evening Snack	Calories	Protein	Carbs	Fiber	Fat	Added Sugar
Time: Totals:						

Daily Totals	Calories	Protein	Carbs	Fiber	Fat	Added Sugar
Totals for all Meals and Snacks:						

Fitness Activity   Time   Duration

_____

_____

Daily Food Log Day:_____ Date:_____

Hours of Sleep Last Night: ☐ 0-2 ☐ 2-4 ☐ 4-6 ☐ 6-8 ☐ 8-10 ☐ 10+

# of 8 oz. glasses of water consumed: ☐ ☐ ☐ ☐ ☐ ☐ ☐ ☐ ☐

Vitamins, Supplements, Medications:

Breakfast	Calories	Protein	Carbs	Fiber	Fat	Added Sugar

Time: _____ Totals: _____

Mid-Morning Snack	Calories	Protein	Carbs	Fiber	Fat	Added Sugar

Time: _____ Totals: _____

Lunch	Calories	Protein	Carbs	Fiber	Fat	Added Sugar

Time: _____ Totals: _____

Mid-Afternoon Snack	Calories	Protein	Carbs	Fiber	Fat	Added Sugar
Time: Totals:						

Dinner	Calories	Protein	Carbs	Fiber	Fat	Added Sugar
Time: Totals:						

Evening Snack	Calories	Protein	Carbs	Fiber	Fat	Added Sugar
Time: Totals:						

Daily Totals	Calories	Protein	Carbs	Fiber	Fat	Added Sugar
Totals for all Meals and Snacks:						

Fitness Activity   Time   Duration

_____

_____

Week 6 Wrap Up

Did you meet your goals for the week?   ☐ Yes   ☐ No

What helped you reach your goals or what kept you from reaching your goals:

_____

_____

_____

_____

How do you feel about that?

_____

_____

_____

_____

How do you feel about yourself?

_____

_____

_____

_____

Looking back on this past week, what about yourself are you the most proud?

_____

_____

Week 7 Goals

What are your goals for next week?

_____

_____

_____

_____

_____

"This one step – choosing a goal and sticking to it – changes everything."

Scott Reed

Daily Food Log   Day:_____   Date:_____

Hours of Sleep Last Night: ☐ 0-2   ☐ 2-4   ☐ 4-6   ☐ 6-8   ☐ 8-10   ☐ 10+

# of 8 oz. glasses of water consumed: ☐ ☐ ☐ ☐ ☐ ☐ ☐ ☐ ☐ ☐

Vitamins, Supplements, Medications:

Breakfast	Calories	Protein	Carbs	Fiber	Fat	Added Sugar
Time: Totals:						

Mid-Morning Snack	Calories	Protein	Carbs	Fiber	Fat	Added Sugar
Time: Totals:						

Lunch	Calories	Protein	Carbs	Fiber	Fat	Added Sugar
Time: Totals:						

Mid-Afternoon Snack	Calories	Protein	Carbs	Fiber	Fat	Added Sugar
Time: Totals:					

Dinner	Calories	Protein	Carbs	Fiber	Fat	Added Sugar
Time: Totals:					

Evening Snack	Calories	Protein	Carbs	Fiber	Fat	Added Sugar
Time: Totals:					

Daily Totals	Calories	Protein	Carbs	Fiber	Fat	Added Sugar
Totals for all Meals and Snacks:					

Fitness Activity　　　　　　　　　　　　Time　　　Duration

Daily Food Log   Day:_____   Date:_____

Hours of Sleep Last Night: ☐ 0-2   ☐ 2-4   ☐ 4-6   ☐ 6-8   ☐ 8-10   ☐ 10+

# of 8 oz. glasses of water consumed: ☐ ☐ ☐ ☐ ☐ ☐ ☐ ☐ ☐ ☐

Vitamins, Supplements, Medications:

Breakfast	Calories	Protein	Carbs	Fiber	Fat	Added Sugar
Time: Totals:						

Mid-Morning Snack	Calories	Protein	Carbs	Fiber	Fat	Added Sugar
Time: Totals:						

Lunch	Calories	Protein	Carbs	Fiber	Fat	Added Sugar
Time: Totals:						

Mid-Afternoon Snack	Calories	Protein	Carbs	Fiber	Fat	Added Sugar
Time: Totals:						

Dinner	Calories	Protein	Carbs	Fiber	Fat	Added Sugar
Time: Totals:						

Evening Snack	Calories	Protein	Carbs	Fiber	Fat	Added Sugar
Time: Totals:						

Daily Totals	Calories	Protein	Carbs	Fiber	Fat	Added Sugar
Totals for all Meals and Snacks:						

Fitness Activity	Time	Duration

Daily Food Log   Day:_____   Date:_____

Hours of Sleep Last Night: ☐ 0-2   ☐ 2-4   ☐ 4-6   ☐ 6-8   ☐ 8-10   ☐ 10+

# of 8 oz. glasses of water consumed: ☐ ☐ ☐ ☐ ☐ ☐ ☐ ☐ ☐

Vitamins, Supplements, Medications:

Breakfast	Calories	Protein	Carbs	Fiber	Fat	Added Sugar
Time: Totals:						

Mid-Morning Snack	Calories	Protein	Carbs	Fiber	Fat	Added Sugar
Time: Totals:						

Lunch	Calories	Protein	Carbs	Fiber	Fat	Added Sugar
Time: Totals:						

Mid-Afternoon Snack	Calories	Protein	Carbs	Fiber	Fat	Added Sugar
Time: Totals:						

Dinner	Calories	Protein	Carbs	Fiber	Fat	Added Sugar
Time: Totals:						

Evening Snack	Calories	Protein	Carbs	Fiber	Fat	Added Sugar
Time: Totals:						

Daily Totals	Calories	Protein	Carbs	Fiber	Fat	Added Sugar
Totals for all Meals and Snacks:						

Fitness Activity   Time   Duration

_____

_____

Daily Food Log   Day:_____   Date:_____

Hours of Sleep Last Night: ☐ 0-2   ☐ 2-4   ☐ 4-6   ☐ 6-8   ☐ 8-10   ☐ 10+

# of 8 oz. glasses of water consumed: ☐ ☐ ☐ ☐ ☐ ☐ ☐ ☐ ☐ ☐

Vitamins, Supplements, Medications:

Breakfast	Calories	Protein	Carbs	Fiber	Fat	Added Sugar

Time: _____   Totals:

Mid-Morning Snack	Calories	Protein	Carbs	Fiber	Fat	Added Sugar

Time: _____   Totals:

Lunch	Calories	Protein	Carbs	Fiber	Fat	Added Sugar

Time: _____   Totals:

Mid-Afternoon Snack

	Calories	Protein	Carbs	Fiber	Fat	Added Sugar
Time: Totals:						

Dinner

	Calories	Protein	Carbs	Fiber	Fat	Added Sugar
Time: Totals:						

Evening Snack

	Calories	Protein	Carbs	Fiber	Fat	Added Sugar
Time: Totals:						

Daily Totals

	Calories	Protein	Carbs	Fiber	Fat	Added Sugar
Totals for all Meals and Snacks:						

Fitness Activity   Time   Duration

_____

_____

Daily Food Log   Day:_____   Date:_____

Hours of Sleep Last Night: ☐ 0-2   ☐ 2-4   ☐ 4-6   ☐ 6-8   ☐ 8-10   ☐ 10+

# of 8 oz. glasses of water consumed: ☐ ☐ ☐ ☐ ☐ ☐ ☐ ☐ ☐ ☐

Vitamins, Supplements, Medications:

Breakfast	Calories	Protein	Carbs	Fiber	Fat	Added Sugar
Time: Totals:						

Mid-Morning Snack	Calories	Protein	Carbs	Fiber	Fat	Added Sugar
Time: Totals:						

Lunch	Calories	Protein	Carbs	Fiber	Fat	Added Sugar
Time: Totals:						

Mid-Afternoon Snack	Calories	Protein	Carbs	Fiber	Fat	Added Sugar
Time: Totals:						

Dinner	Calories	Protein	Carbs	Fiber	Fat	Added Sugar
Time: Totals:						

Evening Snack	Calories	Protein	Carbs	Fiber	Fat	Added Sugar
Time: Totals:						

Daily Totals	Calories	Protein	Carbs	Fiber	Fat	Added Sugar
Totals for all Meals and Snacks:						

Fitness Activity   Time   Duration

_____

_____

Daily Food Log   Day:_____   Date:_____

Hours of Sleep Last Night: ☐ 0-2   ☐ 2-4   ☐ 4-6   ☐ 6-8   ☐ 8-10   ☐ 10+

# of 8 oz. glasses of water consumed: ☐ ☐ ☐ ☐ ☐ ☐ ☐ ☐ ☐ ☐

Vitamins, Supplements, Medications:

Breakfast	Calories	Protein	Carbs	Fiber	Fat	Added Sugar
Time: Totals:						

Mid-Morning Snack	Calories	Protein	Carbs	Fiber	Fat	Added Sugar
Time: Totals:						

Lunch	Calories	Protein	Carbs	Fiber	Fat	Added Sugar
Time: Totals:						

Mid-Afternoon Snack	Calories	Protein	Carbs	Fiber	Fat	Added Sugar
Time: Totals:						

Dinner	Calories	Protein	Carbs	Fiber	Fat	Added Sugar
Time: Totals:						

Evening Snack	Calories	Protein	Carbs	Fiber	Fat	Added Sugar
Time: Totals:						

Daily Totals	Calories	Protein	Carbs	Fiber	Fat	Added Sugar
Totals for all Meals and Snacks:						

Fitness Activity   Time   Duration

Daily Food Log　　　　Day:_____　　　Date:_____

Hours of Sleep Last Night: ☐ 0-2　☐ 2-4　☐ 4-6　☐ 6-8　☐ 8-10　☐ 10+

# of 8 oz. glasses of water consumed: ☐ ☐ ☐ ☐ ☐ ☐ ☐ ☐ ☐ ☐

Vitamins, Supplements, Medications:

Breakfast	Calories	Protein	Carbs	Fiber	Fat	Added Sugar
_____						
_____						
_____						
_____						
Time: _____ Totals: _____						

Mid-Morning Snack	Calories	Protein	Carbs	Fiber	Fat	Added Sugar
_____						
_____						
_____						
Time: _____ Totals: _____						

Lunch	Calories	Protein	Carbs	Fiber	Fat	Added Sugar
_____						
_____						
_____						
_____						
Time: _____ Totals: _____						

Mid-Afternoon Snack	Calories	Protein	Carbs	Fiber	Fat	Added Sugar
Time:　　Totals:						

Dinner	Calories	Protein	Carbs	Fiber	Fat	Added Sugar
Time:　　Totals:						

Evening Snack	Calories	Protein	Carbs	Fiber	Fat	Added Sugar
Time:　　Totals:						

Daily Totals	Calories	Protein	Carbs	Fiber	Fat	Added Sugar
Totals for all Meals and Snacks:						

Fitness Activity　　　　　　　　　　Time　　　Duration

_____

_____

Week 7 Wrap Up

Did you meet your goals for the week?   ☐ Yes   ☐ No

What helped you reach your goals or what kept you from reaching your goals:

_____

_____

_____

_____

How do you feel about that?

_____

_____

_____

_____

How do you feel about yourself?

_____

_____

_____

_____

Looking back on this past week, what about yourself are you the most proud?

_____

_____

Week 8 Goals

What are your goals for next week?

_____

_____

_____

_____

_____

"Success is the child of drudgery and perseverance. It cannot be coaxed or bribed; pay the price and it is yours."

Orison Swett Marden

Daily Food Log   Day:_____   Date:_____

Hours of Sleep Last Night: ☐ 0-2   ☐ 2-4   ☐ 4-6   ☐ 6-8   ☐ 8-10   ☐ 10+

# of 8 oz. glasses of water consumed: ☐ ☐ ☐ ☐ ☐ ☐ ☐ ☐ ☐ ☐

Vitamins, Supplements, Medications:

Breakfast	Calories	Protein	Carbs	Fiber	Fat	Added Sugar
Time: Totals:						

Mid-Morning Snack	Calories	Protein	Carbs	Fiber	Fat	Added Sugar
Time: Totals:						

Lunch	Calories	Protein	Carbs	Fiber	Fat	Added Sugar
Time: Totals:						

Mid-Afternoon Snack

	Calories	Protein	Carbs	Fiber	Fat	Added Sugar

Time: Totals:

Dinner

	Calories	Protein	Carbs	Fiber	Fat	Added Sugar

Time: Totals:

Evening Snack

	Calories	Protein	Carbs	Fiber	Fat	Added Sugar

Time: Totals:

Daily Totals

	Calories	Protein	Carbs	Fiber	Fat	Added Sugar
Totals for all Meals and Snacks:						

Fitness Activity

Time   Duration

Daily Food Log Day:_____ Date:_____

Hours of Sleep Last Night: ☐ 0-2 ☐ 2-4 ☐ 4-6 ☐ 6-8 ☐ 8-10 ☐ 10+

# of 8 oz. glasses of water consumed: ☐ ☐ ☐ ☐ ☐ ☐ ☐ ☐ ☐

Vitamins, Supplements, Medications:

Breakfast	Calories	Protein	Carbs	Fiber	Fat	Added Sugar
Time: Totals:						

Mid-Morning Snack	Calories	Protein	Carbs	Fiber	Fat	Added Sugar
Time: Totals:						

Lunch	Calories	Protein	Carbs	Fiber	Fat	Added Sugar
Time: Totals:						

Mid-Afternoon Snack

	Calories	Protein	Carbs	Fiber	Fat	Added Sugar

Time: Totals:

Dinner

	Calories	Protein	Carbs	Fiber	Fat	Added Sugar

Time: Totals:

Evening Snack

	Calories	Protein	Carbs	Fiber	Fat	Added Sugar

Time: Totals:

Daily Totals

	Calories	Protein	Carbs	Fiber	Fat	Added Sugar
Totals for all Meals and Snacks:						

Fitness Activity   Time   Duration

_____

_____

Daily Food Log Day:_____ Date:_____

Hours of Sleep Last Night: ☐ 0-2 ☐ 2-4 ☐ 4-6 ☐ 6-8 ☐ 8-10 ☐ 10+

# of 8 oz. glasses of water consumed: ☐ ☐ ☐ ☐ ☐ ☐ ☐ ☐ ☐

Vitamins, Supplements, Medications:

Breakfast	Calories	Protein	Carbs	Fiber	Fat	Added Sugar

Time: Totals:

Mid-Morning Snack	Calories	Protein	Carbs	Fiber	Fat	Added Sugar

Time: Totals:

Lunch	Calories	Protein	Carbs	Fiber	Fat	Added Sugar

Time: Totals:

Mid-Afternoon Snack	Calories	Protein	Carbs	Fiber	Fat	Added Sugar
Time: Totals:						

Dinner	Calories	Protein	Carbs	Fiber	Fat	Added Sugar
Time: Totals:						

Evening Snack	Calories	Protein	Carbs	Fiber	Fat	Added Sugar
Time: Totals:						

Daily Totals	Calories	Protein	Carbs	Fiber	Fat	Added Sugar
Totals for all Meals and Snacks:						

Fitness Activity   Time   Duration

_____

_____

Daily Food Log

Day:_____   Date:_____

Hours of Sleep Last Night: ☐ 0-2   ☐ 2-4   ☐ 4-6   ☐ 6-8   ☐ 8-10   ☐ 10+

# of 8 oz. glasses of water consumed: ☐ ☐ ☐ ☐ ☐ ☐ ☐ ☐ ☐

Vitamins, Supplements, Medications:

Breakfast	Calories	Protein	Carbs	Fiber	Fat	Added Sugar
Time: Totals:						

Mid-Morning Snack	Calories	Protein	Carbs	Fiber	Fat	Added Sugar
Time: Totals:						

Lunch	Calories	Protein	Carbs	Fiber	Fat	Added Sugar
Time: Totals:						

Mid-Afternoon Snack	Calories	Protein	Carbs	Fiber	Fat	Added Sugar
Time: Totals:						

Dinner	Calories	Protein	Carbs	Fiber	Fat	Added Sugar
Time: Totals:						

Evening Snack	Calories	Protein	Carbs	Fiber	Fat	Added Sugar
Time: Totals:						

Daily Totals	Calories	Protein	Carbs	Fiber	Fat	Added Sugar
Totals for all Meals and Snacks:						

Fitness Activity   Time   Duration

_____

_____

Daily Food Log Day:_____ Date:_____

Hours of Sleep Last Night: ☐ 0-2   ☐ 2-4   ☐ 4-6   ☐ 6-8   ☐ 8-10   ☐ 10+

# of 8 oz. glasses of water consumed: ☐ ☐ ☐ ☐ ☐ ☐ ☐ ☐ ☐

Vitamins, Supplements, Medications:

Breakfast	Calories	Protein	Carbs	Fiber	Fat	Added Sugar
Time: Totals:						

Mid-Morning Snack	Calories	Protein	Carbs	Fiber	Fat	Added Sugar
Time: Totals:						

Lunch	Calories	Protein	Carbs	Fiber	Fat	Added Sugar
Time: Totals:						

Mid-Afternoon Snack	Calories	Protein	Carbs	Fiber	Fat	Added Sugar
Time: Totals:					

Dinner	Calories	Protein	Carbs	Fiber	Fat	Added Sugar
Time: Totals:					

Evening Snack	Calories	Protein	Carbs	Fiber	Fat	Added Sugar
Time: Totals:					

Daily Totals	Calories	Protein	Carbs	Fiber	Fat	Added Sugar
Totals for all Meals and Snacks:					

Fitness Activity   Time   Duration

_____

_____

Daily Food Log   Day:_____   Date:_____

Hours of Sleep Last Night: ☐ 0-2   ☐ 2-4   ☐ 4-6   ☐ 6-8   ☐ 8-10   ☐ 10+

# of 8 oz. glasses of water consumed: ☐ ☐ ☐ ☐ ☐ ☐ ☐ ☐ ☐

Vitamins, Supplements, Medications:

Breakfast	Calories	Protein	Carbs	Fiber	Fat	Added Sugar
Time: Totals:						

Mid-Morning Snack	Calories	Protein	Carbs	Fiber	Fat	Added Sugar
Time: Totals:						

Lunch	Calories	Protein	Carbs	Fiber	Fat	Added Sugar
Time: Totals:						

Mid-Afternoon Snack	Calories	Protein	Carbs	Fiber	Fat	Added Sugar
Time: Totals:						

Dinner	Calories	Protein	Carbs	Fiber	Fat	Added Sugar
Time: Totals:						

Evening Snack	Calories	Protein	Carbs	Fiber	Fat	Added Sugar
Time: Totals:						

Daily Totals	Calories	Protein	Carbs	Fiber	Fat	Added Sugar
Totals for all Meals and Snacks:						

Fitness Activity   Time   Duration

_____

_____

Daily Food Log   Day:_____   Date:_____

Hours of Sleep Last Night: ☐ 0-2   ☐ 2-4   ☐ 4-6   ☐ 6-8   ☐ 8-10   ☐ 10+

# of 8 oz. glasses of water consumed: ☐ ☐ ☐ ☐ ☐ ☐ ☐ ☐ ☐

Vitamins, Supplements, Medications:

Breakfast	Calories	Protein	Carbs	Fiber	Fat	Added Sugar
Time: Totals:						

Mid-Morning Snack	Calories	Protein	Carbs	Fiber	Fat	Added Sugar
Time: Totals:						

Lunch	Calories	Protein	Carbs	Fiber	Fat	Added Sugar
Time: Totals:						

Mid-Afternoon Snack	Calories	Protein	Carbs	Fiber	Fat	Added Sugar
Time: Totals:						

Dinner	Calories	Protein	Carbs	Fiber	Fat	Added Sugar
Time: Totals:						

Evening Snack	Calories	Protein	Carbs	Fiber	Fat	Added Sugar
Time: Totals:						

Daily Totals	Calories	Protein	Carbs	Fiber	Fat	Added Sugar
Totals for all Meals and Snacks:						

Fitness Activity   Time   Duration

_____

_____

Week 8 Wrap Up

Did you meet your goals for the week? ☐ Yes ☐ No

What helped you reach your goals or what kept you from reaching your goals:

_____

_____

_____

_____

How do you feel about that?

_____

_____

_____

_____

How do you feel about yourself?

_____

_____

_____

_____

Looking back on this past week, what about yourself are you the most proud?

_____

_____

CONGRATULATIONS!

You've completed an 8-week exercise of getting a better idea of what you are eating and when you are eating it. You are developing important habits that put you in charge of your relationship with food and of taking control of your health.

Has your interaction with and attitude towards food changed? ☐ Yes ☐ No

How?

_____

_____

_____

How do you feel about that?

_____

_____

How do you feel about yourself?

_____

_____

Looking back on this past 8 weeks, what about yourself are you the most proud?

_____

_____

If you are committed to continuing on this journey of control and empowerment, we hope you will choose to get another copy of this food log.

Bonus

To say "Thanks" for making a commitment to your good health with this food log, here are two free reports that you might find of interest.

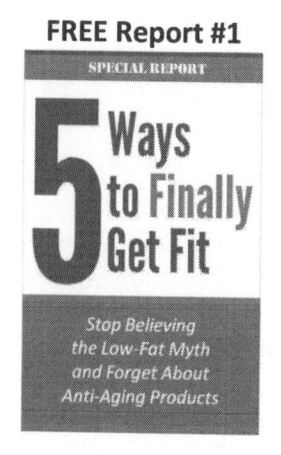

FREE Report #1

To download *"5 Ways to Finally Get Fit"* go to:
http://www.fastforwardpublishing.com/Thank-You-5-Ways-to-Finally-Get-Fti.html

FREE Report #2

To download *"A Nutritional Guide to Fat Loss"* go to
http://www.fastforwardpublishing.com/Thank-You-Nutritional-Guide.html

FastForwardPublishing.com

You might also be interested in one of our "Gratitude Journals" from James Allen Proctor – all available at amazon.com and other retailers:

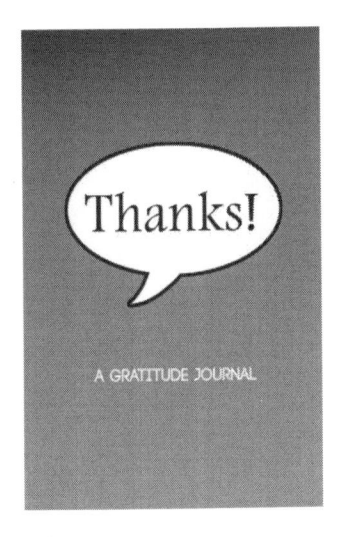

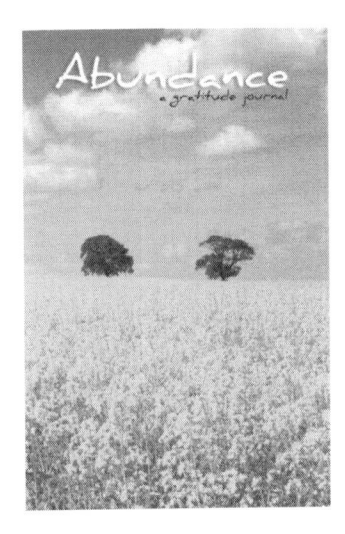

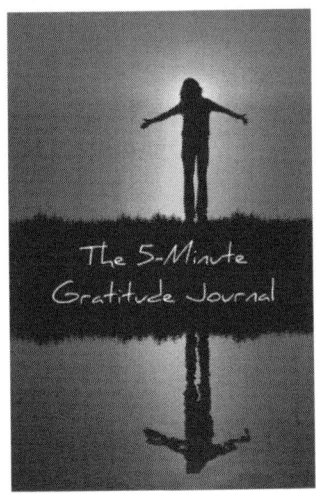

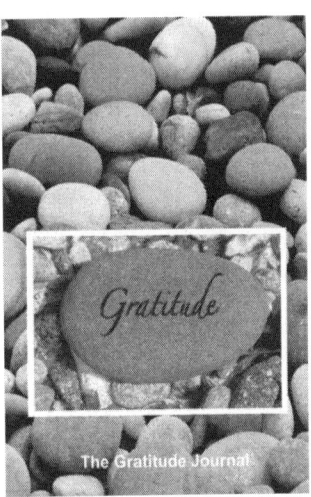

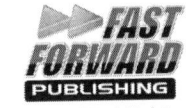

FastForwardPublishing.com

About the Author

Jean LeGrand is best known for his recipe books. He admits that he is unsure whether he cooks because he likes to eat or that he eats because he likes to cook.

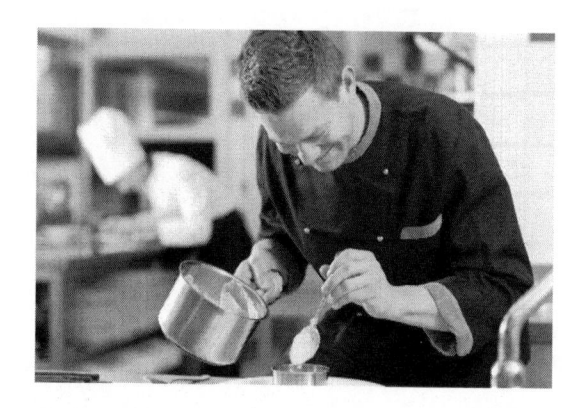

Along with his popular food logs and diet diaries, other books by best-selling author Jean LeGrand include:

Fruit Infused Water Recipes
The Maple Syrup Cookbook Volume 1
The Maple Syrup Cookbook Volume 2
Romantic Treats
Top Paleo Diet Recipes
FrankenFood Recipes #1
FrankenFood Recipes #2
Delicious & Healthy Paleo Recipes
Easter Brunch
Easter Dinner
Mother's Day Recipes
St. Patrick's Day
Irish Dinner
Irish Drinks
Irish Toasts
Irish Treats

All are available at amazon.com and other retailers

Thank you
Can I Ask a Favor?

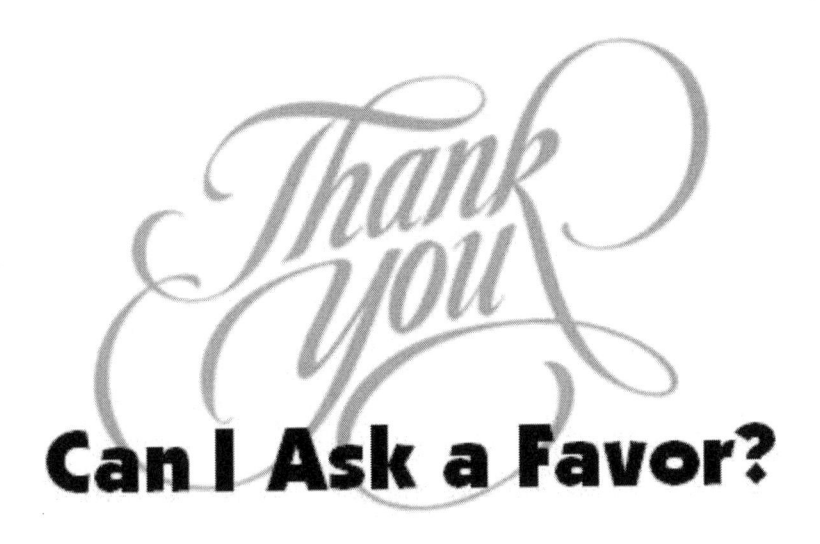

Thank you so much for choosing this journal to help you focus on a healthy lifestyle. I hope it is proving useful and you are well on your way to reaching your goals.

As you probably know, many people look at the reviews on Amazon before they decide to make a purchase.

If you are happy with the value this journal offers, **could you please take a minute to leave a review** with your feedback?

Just go to Amazon.com, look up *Intermittent Fasting Food Log - LeGrand*, go to the book's page) and scroll down until you see the orange "Write a customer review button", click it and write a few words about why you like this product.

A couple of minutes is all I'm asking for, and it would mean the world to me.

Thank you so much,

Jean

14283345R00080

Printed in Great Britain
by Amazon.co.uk, Ltd.,
Marston Gate.